Name of Look

Evening ◯

Daytime ◯

Face

Moisturizer

Concealer

Foundation

Highlight/Blush

Eyes

Brows

Eyelid

Liner

Crease

Mascara

Lips

Liner

Lip Color

Gloss

Notes

Name of Look _______________________

Evening ◯

Daytime ◯

Face

Moisturizer

Concealer

Foundation

Highlight/Blush

Eyes

Brows

Eyelid

Liner

Crease

Mascara

Lips

Liner

Lip Color

Gloss

Notes

Name of Look ______________________

Evening ◯
Daytime ◯

Face

Moisturizer

Concealer

Foundation

Highlight/Blush

Eyes

Brows

Eyelid

Liner

Crease

Mascara

Lips

Liner

Lip Color

Gloss

Notes

Name of Look

Evening ◯
Daytime ◯

Face

Moisturizer

Concealer

Foundation

Highlight/Blush

Eyes

Brows

Eyelid

Liner

Crease

Mascara

Lips

Liner

Lip Color

Gloss

Notes

Name of Look

Evening ◯

Daytime ◯

Face

Moisturizer

Concealer

Foundation

Highlight/Blush

Eyes

Brows

Eyelid

Liner

Crease

Mascara

Lips

Liner

Lip Color

Gloss

Notes

Name of Look ______________________

Evening ◯

Daytime ◯

Face

Moisturizer

Concealer

Foundation

Highlight/Blush

Eyes

Brows

Eyelid

Liner

Crease

Mascara

Lips

Liner

Lip Color

Gloss

Notes

Name of Look

Evening ◯

Daytime ◯

Face

Moisturizer

Concealer

Foundation

Highlight/Blush

Eyes

Brows

Eyelid

Liner

Crease

Mascara

Lips

Liner

Lip Color

Gloss

Notes

Name of Look ___________________

Evening ◯
Daytime ◯

Face

Moisturizer

Concealer

Foundation

Highlight/Blush

Eyes

Brows

Eyelid

Liner

Crease

Mascara

Lips

Liner

Lip Color

Gloss

Notes

Name of Look

Evening ◯

Daytime ◯

Face

Moisturizer

Concealer

Foundation

Highlight/Blush

Eyes

Brows

Eyelid

Liner

Crease

Mascara

Lips

Liner

Lip Color

Gloss

Notes

Name of Look ___________________

Evening ○

Daytime ○

Face

Moisturizer

Concealer

Foundation

Highlight/Blush

Eyes

Brows

Eyelid

Liner

Crease

Mascara

Lips

Liner

Lip Color

Gloss

Notes

Name of Look

Evening ○
Daytime ○

Face

Moisturizer

Concealer

Foundation

Highlight/Blush

Eyes

Brows

Eyelid

Liner

Crease

Mascara

Lips

Liner

Lip Color

Gloss

Notes

Name of Look ________________

Evening ○
Daytime ○

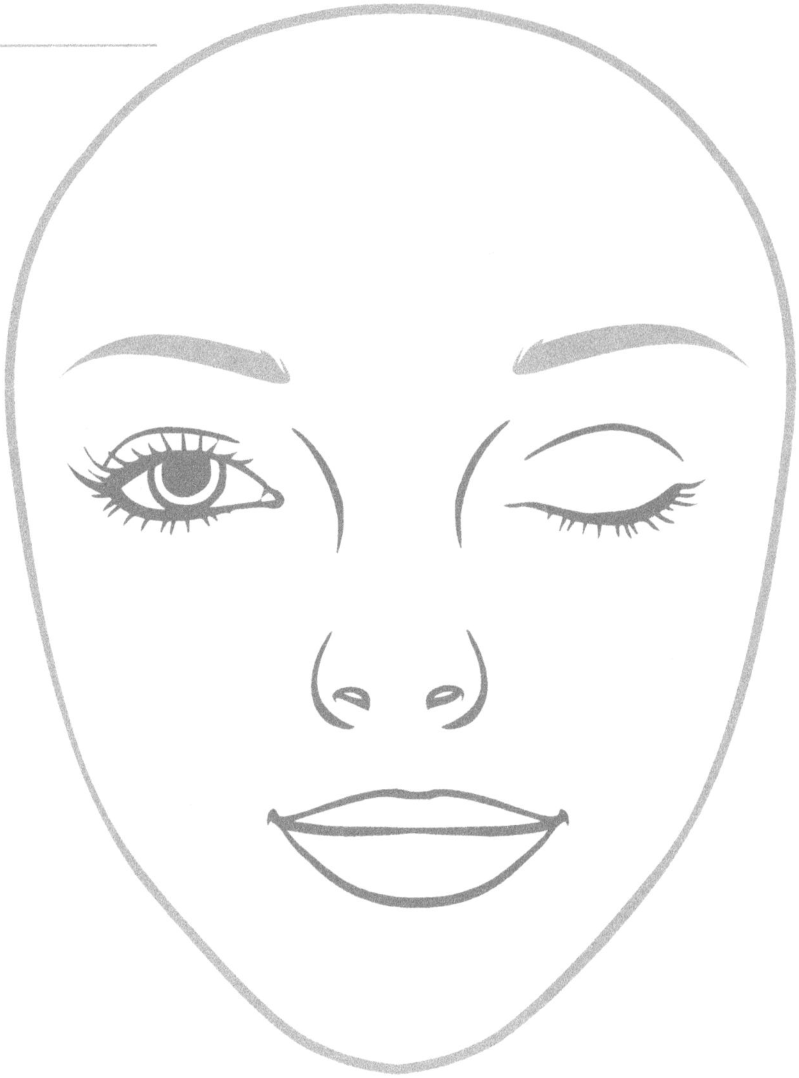

Face

Moisturizer

Concealer

Foundation

Highlight/Blush

Eyes

Brows

Eyelid

Liner

Crease

Mascara

Lips

Liner

Lip Color

Gloss

Notes

Name of Look

Evening ◯

Daytime ◯

Face

Moisturizer

Concealer

Foundation

Highlight/Blush

Eyes

Brows

Eyelid

Liner

Crease

Mascara

Lips

Liner

Lip Color

Gloss

Notes

Name of Look

Evening ◯
Daytime ◯

Face

Moisturizer

Concealer

Foundation

Highlight/Blush

Eyes

Brows

Eyelid

Liner

Crease

Mascara

Lips

Liner

Lip Color

Gloss

Notes

Name of Look ______________________

Evening ○
Daytime ○

Face

Moisturizer

Concealer

Foundation

Highlight/Blush

Eyes

Brows

Eyelid

Liner

Crease

Mascara

Lips

Liner

Lip Color

Gloss

Notes

Name of Look

Evening ◯

Daytime ◯

Face

Moisturizer

Concealer

Foundation

Highlight/Blush

Eyes

Brows

Eyelid

Liner

Crease

Mascara

Lips

Liner

Lip Color

Gloss

Notes

Name of Look

Evening ○
Daytime ○

Face

Moisturizer

Concealer

Foundation

Highlight/Blush

Eyes

Brows

Eyelid

Liner

Crease

Mascara

Lips

Liner

Lip Color

Gloss

Notes

Name of Look ________________

Evening ◯

Daytime ◯

Face

Moisturizer

Concealer

Foundation

Highlight/Blush

Eyes

Brows

Eyelid

Liner

Crease

Mascara

Lips

Liner

Lip Color

Gloss

Notes

Name of Look

Evening ◯

Daytime ◯

Face

Moisturizer

Concealer

Foundation

Highlight/Blush

Eyes

Brows

Eyelid

Liner

Crease

Mascara

Lips

Liner

Lip Color

Gloss

Notes

Name of Look

Evening ◯

Daytime ◯

Face

Moisturizer

Concealer

Foundation

Highlight/Blush

Eyes

Brows

Eyelid

Liner

Crease

Mascara

Lips

Liner

Lip Color

Gloss

Notes

Name of Look

Evening ◯

Daytime ◯

Face

Moisturizer

Concealer

Foundation

Highlight/Blush

Eyes

Brows

Eyelid

Liner

Crease

Mascara

Lips

Liner

Lip Color

Gloss

Notes

Name of Look

Evening ◯

Daytime ◯

Face

Moisturizer

Concealer

Foundation

Highlight/Blush

Eyes

Brows

Eyelid

Liner

Crease

Mascara

Lips

Liner

Lip Color

Gloss

Notes

Name of Look _______________

Evening ◯
Daytime ◯

Face

Moisturizer

Concealer

Foundation

Highlight/Blush

Eyes

Brows

Eyelid

Liner

Crease

Mascara

Lips

Liner

Lip Color

Gloss

Notes

Name of Look ______________________

Evening ○
Daytime ○

Face

Moisturizer

____

Concealer

____

Foundation

____

Highlight/Blush

____

Eyes

Brows

____

Eyelid

____

Liner

____

Crease

____

Mascara

Lips

Liner

____

Lip Color

____

Gloss

Notes

Name of Look ______________________

Evening ◯
Daytime ◯

Face

Moisturizer

Concealer

Foundation

Highlight/Blush

Eyes

Brows

Eyelid

Liner

Crease

Mascara

Lips

Liner

Lip Color

Gloss

Notes

Name of Look _______________

Evening ○
Daytime ○

Face

Moisturizer

Concealer

Foundation

Highlight/Blush

Eyes

Brows

Eyelid

Liner

Crease

Mascara

Lips

Liner

Lip Color

Gloss

Notes

Name of Look

Evening ◯

Daytime ◯

Face

Moisturizer

Concealer

Foundation

Highlight/Blush

Eyes

Brows

Eyelid

Liner

Crease

Mascara

Lips

Liner

Lip Color

Gloss

Notes

Name of Look ________________

Evening ◯
Daytime ◯

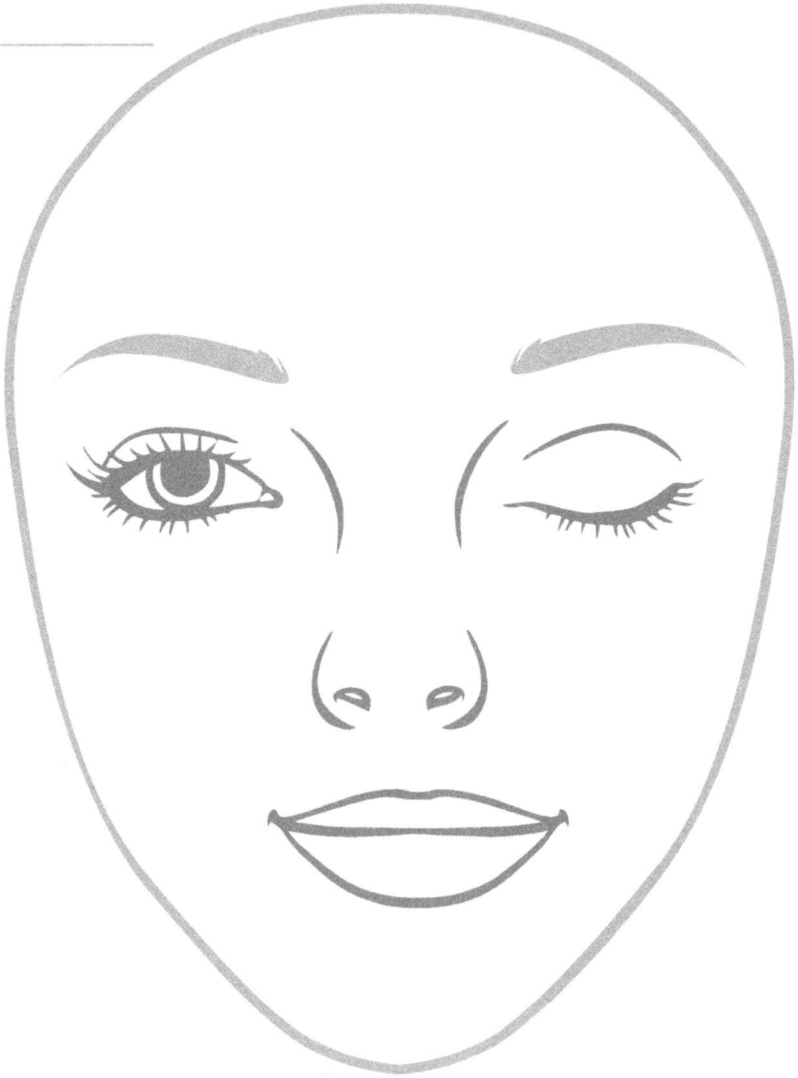

Face

Moisturizer

Concealer

Foundation

Highlight/Blush

Eyes

Brows

Eyelid

Liner

Crease

Mascara

Lips

Liner

Lip Color

Gloss

Notes

Name of Look ________________________

Evening ◯

Daytime ◯

Face

Moisturizer

Concealer

Foundation

Highlight/Blush

Eyes

Brows

Eyelid

Liner

Crease

Mascara

Lips

Liner

Lip Color

Gloss

Notes

Name of Look _______________

Evening ○
Daytime ○

Face

Moisturizer

Concealer

Foundation

Highlight/Blush

Eyes

Brows

Eyelid

Liner

Crease

Mascara

Lips

Liner

Lip Color

Gloss

Notes

Name of Look

Evening ○
Daytime ○

Face

Moisturizer

Concealer

Foundation

Highlight/Blush

Eyes

Brows

Eyelid

Liner

Crease

Mascara

Lips

Liner

Lip Color

Gloss

Notes

Name of Look

Evening ○
Daytime ○

Face

Moisturizer

Concealer

Foundation

Highlight/Blush

Eyes

Brows

Eyelid

Liner

Crease

Mascara

Lips

Liner

Lip Color

Gloss

Notes

Name of Look

Evening ◯

Daytime ◯

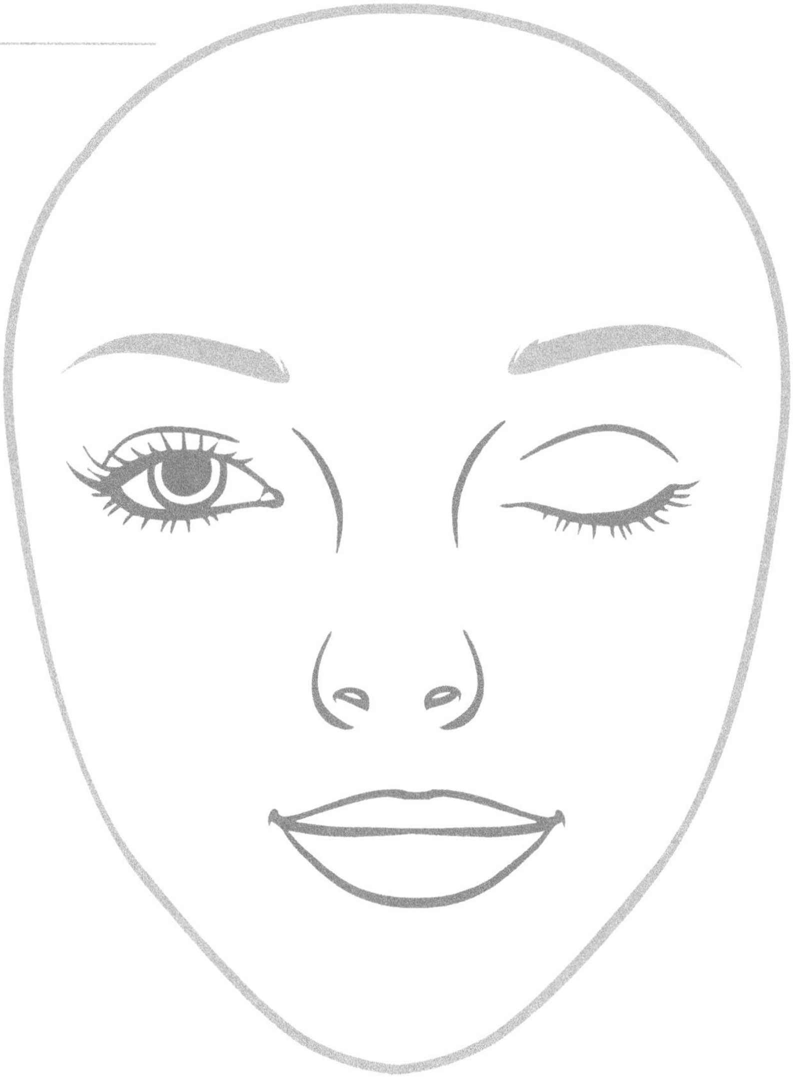

Face

Moisturizer

Concealer

Foundation

Highlight/Blush

Eyes

Brows

Eyelid

Liner

Crease

Mascara

Lips

Liner

Lip Color

Gloss

Notes

Name of Look

Evening ◯

Daytime ◯

Face

Moisturizer

Concealer

Foundation

Highlight/Blush

Eyes

Brows

Eyelid

Liner

Crease

Mascara

Lips

Liner

Lip Color

Gloss

Notes

Name of Look ___________________

Evening ○

Daytime ○

Face

Moisturizer

Concealer

Foundation

Highlight/Blush

Eyes

Brows

Eyelid

Liner

Crease

Mascara

Lips

Liner

Lip Color

Gloss

Notes

Name of Look

Evening ◯
Daytime ◯

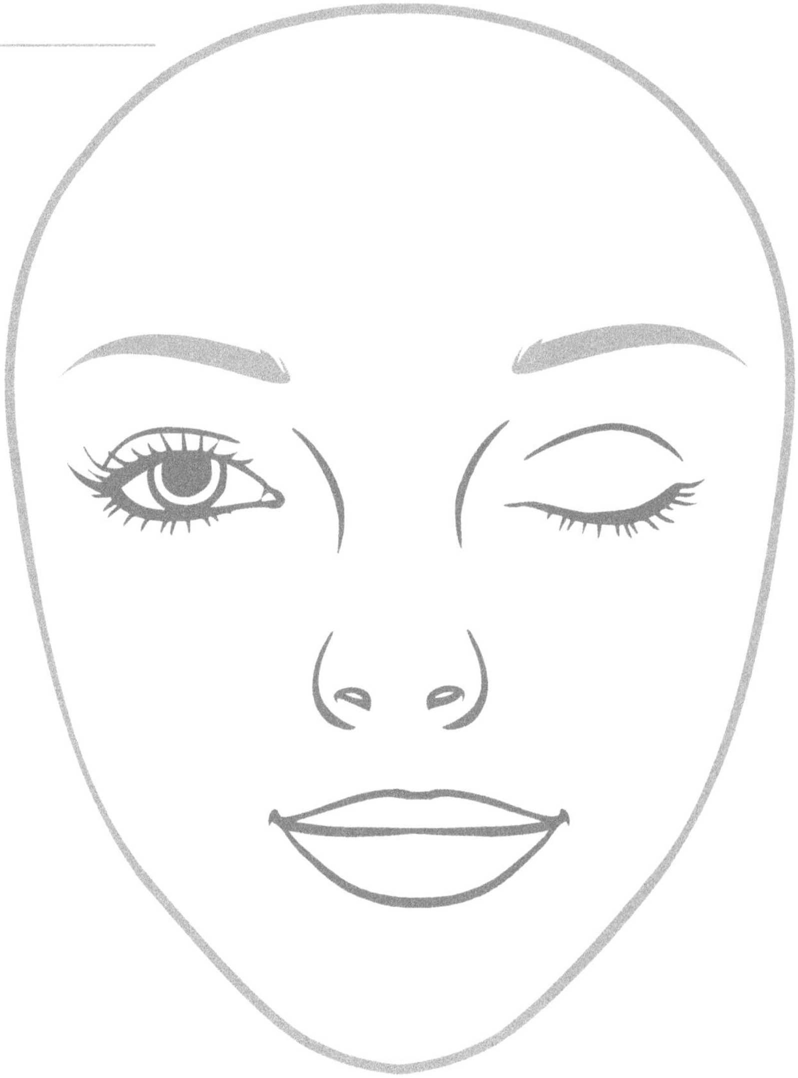

Face

Moisturizer

Concealer

Foundation

Highlight/Blush

Eyes

Brows

Eyelid

Liner

Crease

Mascara

Lips

Liner

Lip Color

Gloss

Notes

Name of Look _______________

Evening ○
Daytime ○

Face

Moisturizer

Concealer

Foundation

Highlight/Blush

Eyes

Brows

Eyelid

Liner

Crease

Mascara

Lips

Liner

Lip Color

Gloss

Notes

Name of Look _______________

Evening ◯

Daytime ◯

Face

Moisturizer

Concealer

Foundation

Highlight/Blush

Eyes

Brows

Eyelid

Liner

Crease

Mascara

Lips

Liner

Lip Color

Gloss

Notes

Name of Look

Evening ⚪

Daytime ⚪

Face

Moisturizer

Concealer

Foundation

Highlight/Blush

Eyes

Brows

Eyelid

Liner

Crease

Mascara

Lips

Liner

Lip Color

Gloss

Notes

Name of Look ______________________

Evening ○
Daytime ○

Face

Moisturizer

Concealer

Foundation

Highlight/Blush

Eyes

Brows

Eyelid

Liner

Crease

Mascara

Lips

Liner

Lip Color

Gloss

Notes

Name of Look

Evening ◯
Daytime ◯

Face

Moisturizer

Concealer

Foundation

Highlight/Blush

Eyes

Brows

Eyelid

Liner

Crease

Mascara

Lips

Liner

Lip Color

Gloss

Notes

Name of Look ___________________

Evening ○

Daytime ○

Face

Moisturizer

Concealer

Foundation

Highlight/Blush

Eyes

Brows

Eyelid

Liner

Crease

Mascara

Lips

Liner

Lip Color

Gloss

Notes

Name of Look

Evening ◯
Daytime ◯

Face

Moisturizer

Concealer

Foundation

Highlight/Blush

Eyes

Brows

Eyelid

Liner

Crease

Mascara

Lips

Liner

Lip Color

Gloss

Notes

Name of Look _______________

Evening ◯

Daytime ◯

Face

Moisturizer

Concealer

Foundation

Highlight/Blush

Eyes

Brows

Eyelid

Liner

Crease

Mascara

Lips

Liner

Lip Color

Gloss

Notes

Name of Look _______________

Evening ◯

Daytime ◯

Face

Moisturizer

Concealer

Foundation

Highlight/Blush

Eyes

Brows

Eyelid

Liner

Crease

Mascara

Lips

Liner

Lip Color

Gloss

Notes

Name of Look ____________________

Evening ○

Daytime ○

Face

Moisturizer

Concealer

Foundation

Highlight/Blush

Eyes

Brows

Eyelid

Liner

Crease

Mascara

Lips

Liner

Lip Color

Gloss

Notes

Name of Look ________________

Evening ◯
Daytime ◯

Face

Moisturizer

Concealer

Foundation

Highlight/Blush

Eyes

Brows

Eyelid

Liner

Crease

Mascara

Lips

Liner

Lip Color

Gloss

Notes

Name of Look _______________________

Evening ◯
Daytime ◯

Face

Moisturizer

Concealer

Foundation

Highlight/Blush

Eyes

Brows

Eyelid

Liner

Crease

Mascara

Lips

Liner

Lip Color

Gloss

Notes

Name of Look

Evening ○
Daytime ○

Face

Moisturizer

Concealer

Foundation

Highlight/Blush

Eyes

Brows

Eyelid

Liner

Crease

Mascara

Lips

Liner

Lip Color

Gloss

Notes

Name of Look _______________

Evening ⭘

Daytime ⭘

Face

Moisturizer

Concealer

Foundation

Highlight/Blush

Eyes

Brows

Eyelid

Liner

Crease

Mascara

Lips

Liner

Lip Color

Gloss

Notes

Name of Look ______________________

Evening ◯

Daytime ◯

Face

Moisturizer

Concealer

Foundation

Highlight/Blush

Eyes

Brows

Eyelid

Liner

Crease

Mascara

Lips

Liner

Lip Color

Gloss

Notes

Name of Look

Evening ◯

Daytime ◯

Face

Moisturizer

Concealer

Foundation

Highlight/Blush

Eyes

Brows

Eyelid

Liner

Crease

Mascara

Lips

Liner

Lip Color

Gloss

Notes

Name of Look

Evening ○
Daytime ○

Face

Moisturizer

Concealer

Foundation

Highlight/Blush

Eyes

Brows

Eyelid

Liner

Crease

Mascara

Lips

Liner

Lip Color

Gloss

Notes

Name of Look

Evening ○
Daytime ○

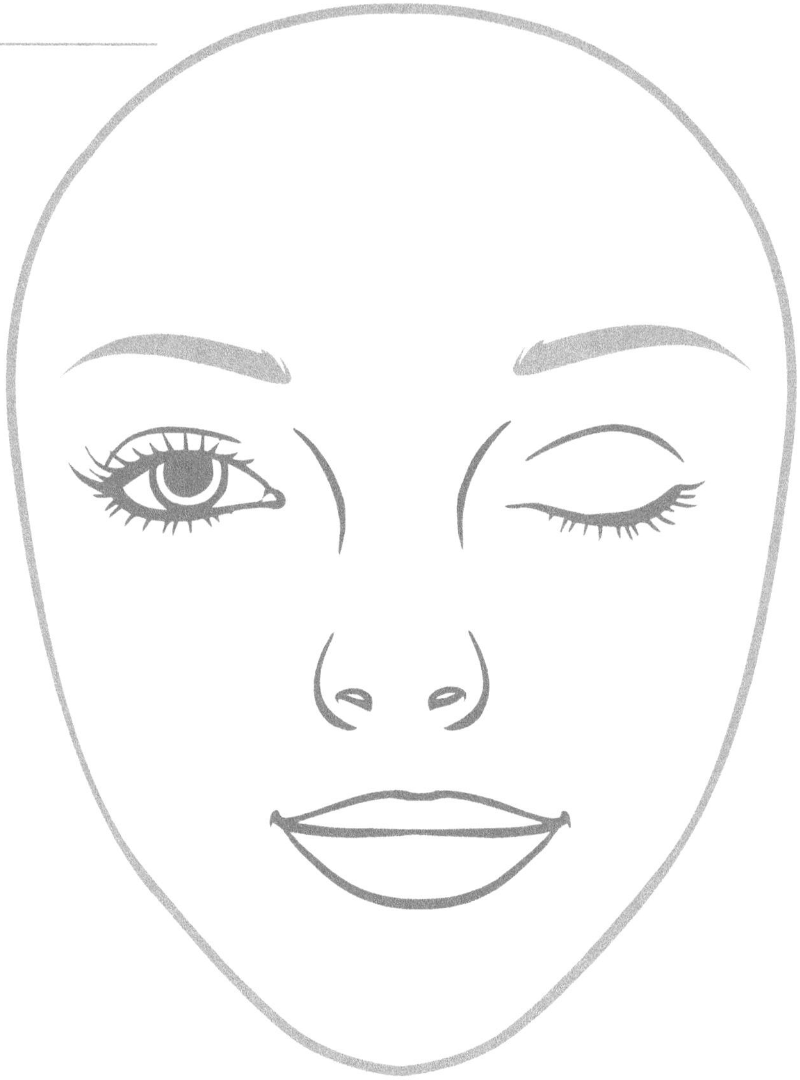

Face

Moisturizer

Concealer

Foundation

Highlight/Blush

Eyes

Brows

Eyelid

Liner

Crease

Mascara

Lips

Liner

Lip Color

Gloss

Notes

Name of Look

Evening ◯

Daytime ◯

Face

Moisturizer

Concealer

Foundation

Highlight/Blush

Eyes

Brows

Eyelid

Liner

Crease

Mascara

Lips

Liner

Lip Color

Gloss

Notes

Name of Look _______________

Evening ◯
Daytime ◯

Face

Moisturizer

Concealer

Foundation

Highlight/Blush

Eyes

Brows

Eyelid

Liner

Crease

Mascara

Lips

Liner

Lip Color

Gloss

Notes

Name of Look

Evening ○
Daytime ○

Face

Moisturizer

Concealer

Foundation

Highlight/Blush

Eyes

Brows

Eyelid

Liner

Crease

Mascara

Lips

Liner

Lip Color

Gloss

Notes

Name of Look ______________________

Evening ◯

Daytime ◯

Face

Moisturizer

Concealer

Foundation

Highlight/Blush

Eyes

Brows

Eyelid

Liner

Crease

Mascara

Lips

Liner

Lip Color

Gloss

Notes

Name of Look

Evening ◯

Daytime ◯

Face

Moisturizer

Concealer

Foundation

Highlight/Blush

Eyes

Brows

Eyelid

Liner

Crease

Mascara

Lips

Liner

Lip Color

Gloss

Notes

Name of Look

____

Evening ○
Daytime ○

Face

Moisturizer

____

Concealer

____

Foundation

____

Highlight/Blush

____

Eyes

Brows

____

Eyelid

____

Liner

____

Crease

____

Mascara

Lips

Liner

____

Lip Color

____

Gloss

Notes

Name of Look

Evening ○
Daytime ○

Face

Moisturizer

Concealer

Foundation

Highlight/Blush

Eyes

Brows

Eyelid

Liner

Crease

Mascara

Lips

Liner

Lip Color

Gloss

Notes

Name of Look ___________________

Evening ⃝
Daytime ⃝

Face

Moisturizer

Concealer

Foundation

Highlight/Blush

Eyes

Brows

Eyelid

Liner

Crease

Mascara

Lips

Liner

Lip Color

Gloss

Notes

Name of Look ___________________

Evening ◯

Daytime ◯

Face

Moisturizer

____

Concealer

____

Foundation

____

Highlight/Blush

____

Eyes

Brows

____

Eyelid

____

Liner

____

Crease

____

Mascara

Lips

Liner

____

Lip Color

____

Gloss

Notes

Name of Look

Evening ⭕
Daytime ⭕

Face

Moisturizer

Concealer

Foundation

Highlight/Blush

Eyes

Brows

Eyelid

Liner

Crease

Mascara

Lips

Liner

Lip Color

Gloss

Notes

Name of Look ___________________

Evening ○
Daytime ○

Face

Moisturizer

Concealer

Foundation

Highlight/Blush

Eyes

Brows

Eyelid

Liner

Crease

Mascara

Lips

Liner

Lip Color

Gloss

Notes

Name of Look ______________________

Evening ◯

Daytime ◯

Face

Moisturizer

Concealer

Foundation

Highlight/Blush

Eyes

Brows

Eyelid

Liner

Crease

Mascara

Lips

Liner

Lip Color

Gloss

Notes

Name of Look

Evening ○

Daytime ○

Face

Moisturizer

Concealer

Foundation

Highlight/Blush

Eyes

Brows

Eyelid

Liner

Crease

Mascara

Lips

Liner

Lip Color

Gloss

Notes

Name of Look

Evening ○
Daytime ○

Face

Moisturizer

Concealer

Foundation

Highlight/Blush

Eyes

Brows

Eyelid

Liner

Crease

Mascara

Lips

Liner

Lip Color

Gloss

Notes

Name of Look

Evening ○
Daytime ○

Face

Moisturizer

Concealer

Foundation

Highlight/Blush

Eyes

Brows

Eyelid

Liner

Crease

Mascara

Lips

Liner

Lip Color

Gloss

Notes

Name of Look ______________________

Evening ◯
Daytime ◯

Face

Moisturizer

Concealer

Foundation

Highlight/Blush

Eyes

Brows

Eyelid

Liner

Crease

Mascara

Lips

Liner

Lip Color

Gloss

Notes

Name of Look ________________________

Evening ◯

Daytime ◯

Face

Moisturizer

Concealer

Foundation

Highlight/Blush

Eyes

Brows

Eyelid

Liner

Crease

Mascara

Lips

Liner

Lip Color

Gloss

Notes

Name of Look ___________________________

Evening ◯

Daytime ◯

Face

Moisturizer

Concealer

Foundation

Highlight/Blush

Eyes

Brows

Eyelid

Liner

Crease

Mascara

Lips

Liner

Lip Color

Gloss

Notes

Name of Look

Evening ◯

Daytime ◯

Face

Moisturizer

Concealer

Foundation

Highlight/Blush

Eyes

Brows

Eyelid

Liner

Crease

Mascara

Lips

Liner

Lip Color

Gloss

Notes

Name of Look

Evening ○
Daytime ○

Face

Moisturizer

Concealer

Foundation

Highlight/Blush

Eyes

Brows

Eyelid

Liner

Crease

Mascara

Lips

Liner

Lip Color

Gloss

Notes

Name of Look

Evening ○
Daytime ○

Face

Moisturizer

Concealer

Foundation

Highlight/Blush

Eyes

Brows

Eyelid

Liner

Crease

Mascara

Lips

Liner

Lip Color

Gloss

Notes

Name of Look ______________________

Evening ⬤

Daytime ⬤

Face

Moisturizer

Concealer

Foundation

Highlight/Blush

Eyes

Brows

Eyelid

Liner

Crease

Mascara

Lips

Liner

Lip Color

Gloss

Notes

Name of Look

Evening ○
Daytime ○

Face

Moisturizer

Concealer

Foundation

Highlight/Blush

Eyes

Brows

Eyelid

Liner

Crease

Mascara

Lips

Liner

Lip Color

Gloss

Notes

Name of Look

Evening ◯

Daytime ◯

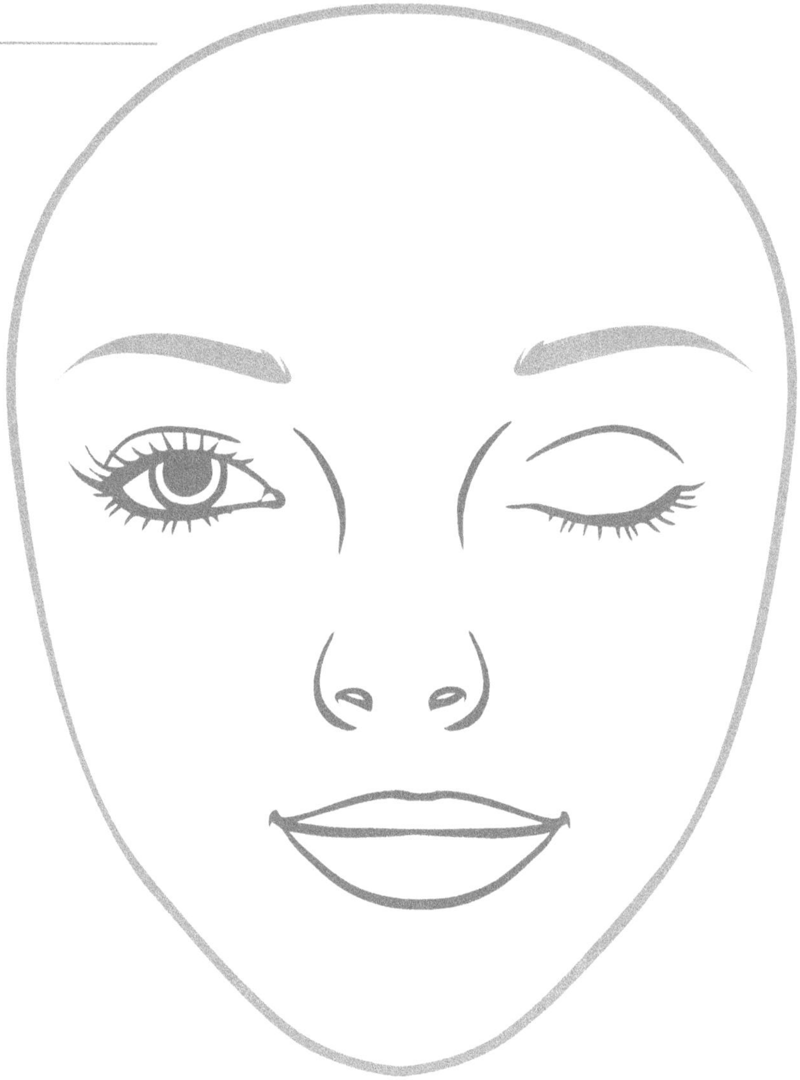

Face

Moisturizer

Concealer

Foundation

Highlight/Blush

Eyes

Brows

Eyelid

Liner

Crease

Mascara

Lips

Liner

Lip Color

Gloss

Notes

Name of Look

Evening ○

Daytime ○

Face

Moisturizer

Concealer

Foundation

Highlight/Blush

Eyes

Brows

Eyelid

Liner

Crease

Mascara

Lips

Liner

Lip Color

Gloss

Notes

Name of Look ___________________

Evening ◯

Daytime ◯

Face

Moisturizer

Concealer

Foundation

Highlight/Blush

Eyes

Brows

Eyelid

Liner

Crease

Mascara

Lips

Liner

Lip Color

Gloss

Notes

Name of Look

Evening ◯
Daytime ◯

Face

Moisturizer

Concealer

Foundation

Highlight/Blush

Eyes

Brows

Eyelid

Liner

Crease

Mascara

Lips

Liner

Lip Color

Gloss

Notes

Name of Look _______________________

Evening ⭘

Daytime ⭘

Face

Moisturizer

Concealer

Foundation

Highlight/Blush

Eyes

Brows

Eyelid

Liner

Crease

Mascara

Lips

Liner

Lip Color

Gloss

Notes

Name of Look

Evening ○
Daytime ○

Face

Moisturizer

Concealer

Foundation

Highlight/Blush

Eyes

Brows

Eyelid

Liner

Crease

Mascara

Lips

Liner

Lip Color

Gloss

Notes

Name of Look

Evening ○
Daytime ○

Face

Moisturizer

Concealer

Foundation

Highlight/Blush

Eyes

Brows

Eyelid

Liner

Crease

Mascara

Lips

Liner

Lip Color

Gloss

Notes

Name of Look

Evening ○

Daytime ○

Face

Moisturizer

Concealer

Foundation

Highlight/Blush

Eyes

Brows

Eyelid

Liner

Crease

Mascara

Lips

Liner

Lip Color

Gloss

Notes

Name of Look ______________________

Evening ○
Daytime ○

Face

Moisturizer

Concealer

Foundation

Highlight/Blush

Eyes

Brows

Eyelid

Liner

Crease

Mascara

Lips

Liner

Lip Color

Gloss

Notes

Name of Look _______________

Evening ◯

Daytime ◯

Face

Moisturizer

Concealer

Foundation

Highlight/Blush

Eyes

Brows

Eyelid

Liner

Crease

Mascara

Lips

Liner

Lip Color

Gloss

Notes

Name of Look ___________________________

Evening ◯

Daytime ◯

Face

Moisturizer

Concealer

Foundation

Highlight/Blush

Eyes

Brows

Eyelid

Liner

Crease

Mascara

Lips

Liner

Lip Color

Gloss

Notes

Name of Look ______________________

Evening ◯
Daytime ◯

Face

Moisturizer

Concealer

Foundation

Highlight/Blush

Eyes

Brows

Eyelid

Liner

Crease

Mascara

Lips

Liner

Lip Color

Gloss

Notes

Name of Look ______________________

Evening ◯
Daytime ◯

Face

Moisturizer

Concealer

Foundation

Highlight/Blush

Eyes

Brows

Eyelid

Liner

Crease

Mascara

Lips

Liner

Lip Color

Gloss

Notes

Name of Look ___________________

Evening ⚪

Daytime ⚪

Face

Moisturizer

Concealer

Foundation

Highlight/Blush

Eyes

Brows

Eyelid

Liner

Crease

Mascara

Lips

Liner

Lip Color

Gloss

Notes

Name of Look ______________________________

Evening ◯

Daytime ◯

Face

Moisturizer

Concealer

Foundation

Highlight/Blush

Eyes

Brows

Eyelid

Liner

Crease

Mascara

Lips

Liner

Lip Color

Gloss

Notes

Name of Look

Evening ◯
Daytime ◯

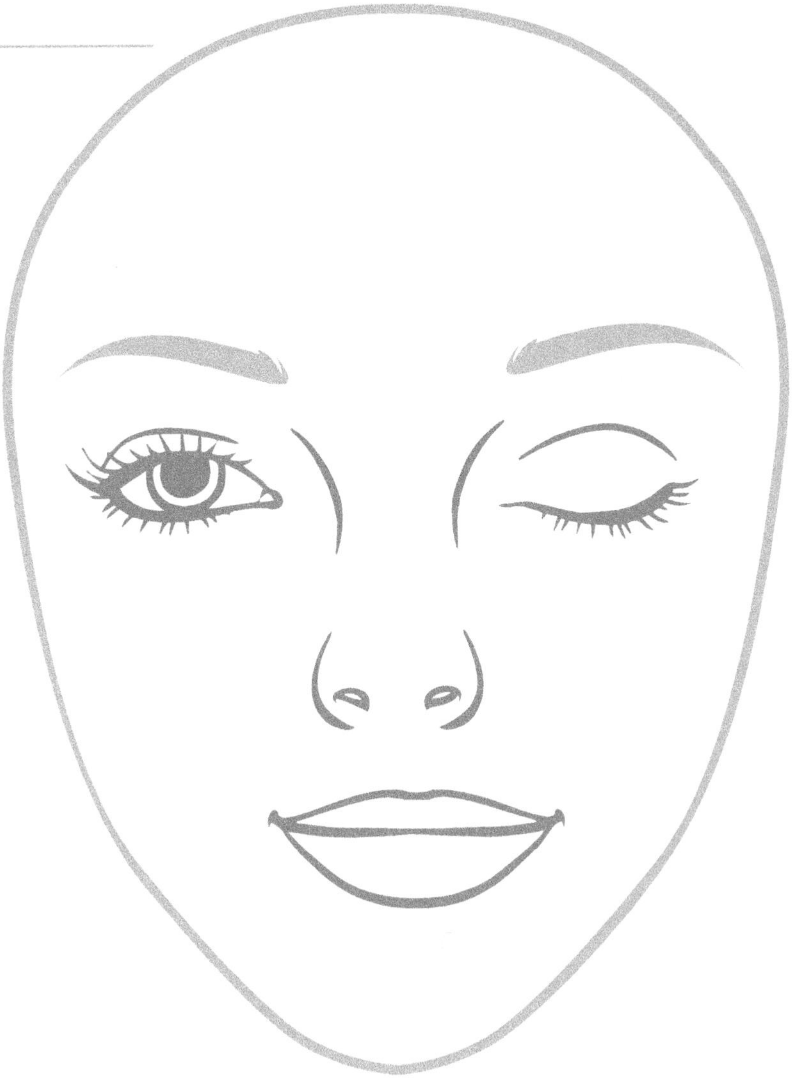

Face

Moisturizer

Concealer

Foundation

Highlight/Blush

Eyes

Brows

Eyelid

Liner

Crease

Mascara

Lips

Liner

Lip Color

Gloss

Notes

Name of Look ______________________

Evening ○

Daytime ○

Face

Moisturizer

Concealer

Foundation

Highlight/Blush

Eyes

Brows

Eyelid

Liner

Crease

Mascara

Lips

Liner

Lip Color

Gloss

Notes

Name of Look

Evening ○

Daytime ○

Face

Moisturizer

Concealer

Foundation

Highlight/Blush

Eyes

Brows

Eyelid

Liner

Crease

Mascara

Lips

Liner

Lip Color

Gloss

Notes

Name of Look ________________

Evening ◯
Daytime ◯

Face

Moisturizer

Concealer

Foundation

Highlight/Blush

Eyes

Brows

Eyelid

Liner

Crease

Mascara

Lips

Liner

Lip Color

Gloss

Notes

Name of Look

Evening ◯
Daytime ◯

Face

Moisturizer

Concealer

Foundation

Highlight/Blush

Eyes

Brows

Eyelid

Liner

Crease

Mascara

Lips

Liner

Lip Color

Gloss

Notes

Name of Look ___________________________

Evening ○

Daytime ○

Face

Moisturizer

Concealer

Foundation

Highlight/Blush

Eyes

Brows

Eyelid

Liner

Crease

Mascara

Lips

Liner

Lip Color

Gloss

Notes

Name of Look

Evening ○

Daytime ○

Face

Moisturizer

Concealer

Foundation

Highlight/Blush

Eyes

Brows

Eyelid

Liner

Crease

Mascara

Lips

Liner

Lip Color

Gloss

Notes

Name of Look _______________

Evening ○

Daytime ○

Face

Moisturizer

Concealer

Foundation

Highlight/Blush

Eyes

Brows

Eyelid

Liner

Crease

Mascara

Lips

Liner

Lip Color

Gloss

Notes

Name of Look _______________

Evening ◯
Daytime ◯

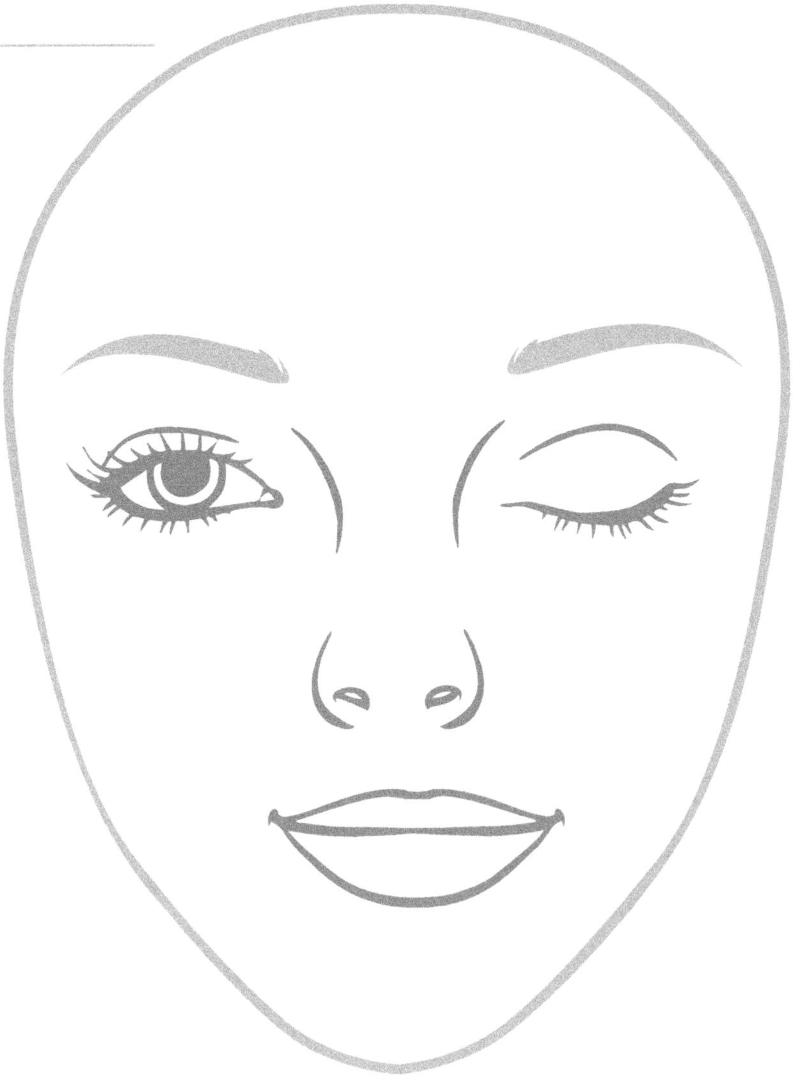

Face

Moisturizer

Concealer

Foundation

Highlight/Blush

Eyes

Brows

Eyelid

Liner

Crease

Mascara

Lips

Liner

Lip Color

Gloss

Notes

Name of Look

Evening ○
Daytime ○

Face

Moisturizer

Concealer

Foundation

Highlight/Blush

Eyes

Brows

Eyelid

Liner

Crease

Mascara

Lips

Liner

Lip Color

Gloss

Notes

Name of Look

Evening ○

Daytime ○

Face

Moisturizer

Concealer

Foundation

Highlight/Blush

Eyes

Brows

Eyelid

Liner

Crease

Mascara

Lips

Liner

Lip Color

Gloss

Notes

Name of Look

Evening ⬭
Daytime ⬭

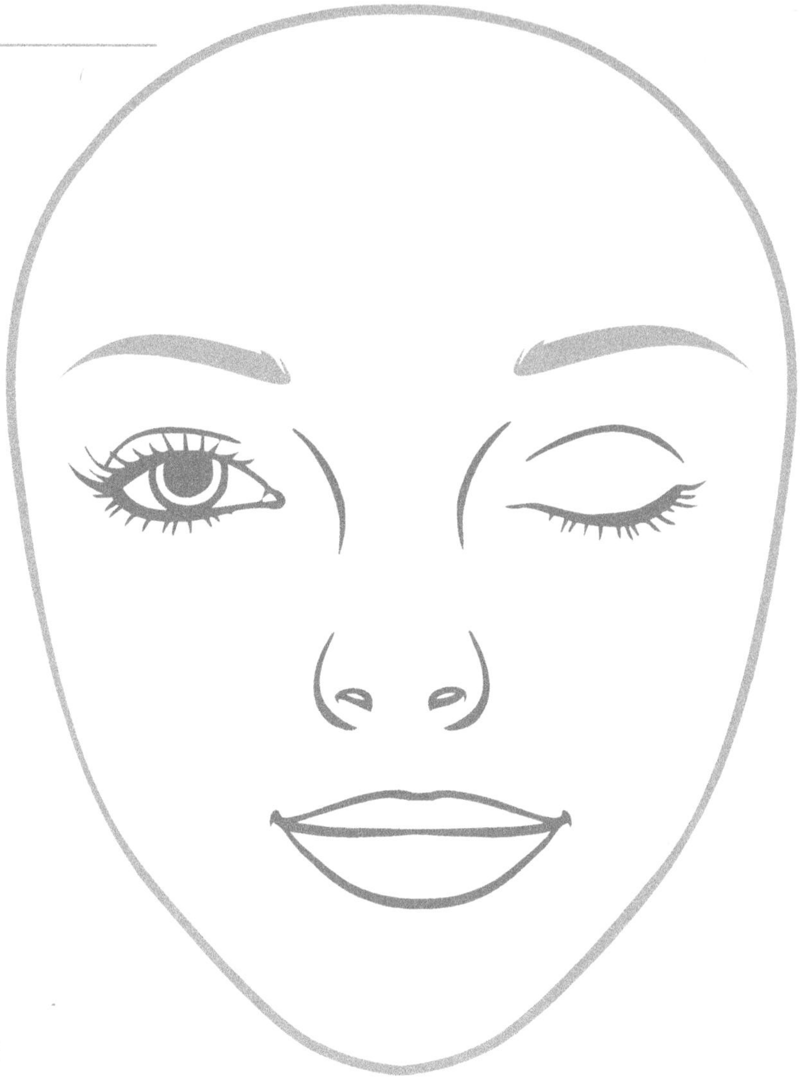

Face

Moisturizer

Concealer

Foundation

Highlight/Blush

Eyes

Brows

Eyelid

Liner

Crease

Mascara

Lips

Liner

Lip Color

Gloss

Notes

Name of Look

Evening ◯
Daytime ◯

Face

Moisturizer

Concealer

Foundation

Highlight/Blush

Eyes

Brows

Eyelid

Liner

Crease

Mascara

Lips

Liner

Lip Color

Gloss

Notes

Name of Look

Evening ◯

Daytime ◯

Face

Moisturizer

Concealer

Foundation

Highlight/Blush

Eyes

Brows

Eyelid

Liner

Crease

Mascara

Lips

Liner

Lip Color

Gloss

Notes

Name of Look

Evening ◯
Daytime ◯

Face

Moisturizer

Concealer

Foundation

Highlight/Blush

Eyes

Brows

Eyelid

Liner

Crease

Mascara

Lips

Liner

Lip Color

Gloss

Notes

Name of Look

Evening ○
Daytime ○

Face

Moisturizer

Concealer

Foundation

Highlight/Blush

Eyes

Brows

Eyelid

Liner

Crease

Mascara

Lips

Liner

Lip Color

Gloss

Notes

Name of Look

Evening ◯
Daytime ◯

Face

Moisturizer

Concealer

Foundation

Highlight/Blush

Eyes

Brows

Eyelid

Liner

Crease

Mascara

Lips

Liner

Lip Color

Gloss

Notes

Name of Look _______________

Evening ◯

Daytime ◯

Face

Moisturizer

Concealer

Foundation

Highlight/Blush

Eyes

Brows

Eyelid

Liner

Crease

Mascara

Lips

Liner

Lip Color

Gloss

Notes

www.ingramcontent.com/pod-product-compliance
Lightning Source LLC
Chambersburg PA
CBHW081346160726
48000CB00010B/3246